CORE STRENGTH

TRAINING MANUAL

Unlock Your Power, Master Core Strength Training Techniques For Stability In Your Fitness Regimen, Enthusiasts And Athletes

LAMBERT FETTERMAN

DISCLAIMER

The content in this book is offered only for general informative purposes. While every effort has been taken to guarantee the content's accuracy and completeness, the author and publisher accept no responsibility for any mistakes or omissions, or for the results of using the information given herein. The methods, recommendations, and directions in this book are not guaranteed to be appropriate for every person, and readers should exercise caution and seek professional counsel if required before undertaking any of the projects or techniques detailed in this book.

Table of Contents

INTRODUCTION

Explaining The Importance Of Core Strength

Core muscles are essential for body stabilization, movement facilitation, and posture maintenance. They serve as the foundation for practically every action the body does, from basic everyday duties to major sporting pursuits. The core is made up of more than just the abdominal muscles; it also includes the pelvis, lower back, and hips, all of which work together to give stability and strength.

A strong core has various advantages, including:

1. **Stability and balance:** Core strength promotes stability, lowering the chance of falling or injuring oneself while moving.

2. **Enhancement of Posture:** A strong core helps to maintain excellent posture, minimizing pain and possible spinal disorders.

3. With a stabilized core, daily tasks such as bending, lifting, and reaching become more efficient.

4. **Athletic Performance:** Athletes in a variety of sports depend on a strong core to generate power and perform well.

5. **Injury Prevention:** A strong core lowers the incidence of back problems and muscular strains.

Brief Overview Of Core Muscles

Understanding the core muscles is critical when exercising for core strength. It is not only about the surface abdominal muscles; deeper levels are also involved:

1. Rectus Abdominis: Known colloquially as the six-pack muscles, they are the superficial abdominal muscles that aid in trunk flexion.

2. Transverse Abdominis: A deep abdominal muscle that acts like a corset, giving spine stability and internal organ support.

3. Obliques are muscles on the sides of the abdomen that allow for twisting and bending actions.

4. **Erector Spinae:** These muscles go down the spine and help to maintain the spine upright.

5. **Multifidus:** Deep muscles that run the length of the spine and support and rotate the vertebrae.

Methods Of Core Strength Training

Core strength is more than simply doing crunches all day. A range of exercises targeting distinct core muscles, such as stability, rotation, flexion, and extension motions, are used in effective training.

To gain comprehensive core strength, use a variety of workouts such as planks, bridges, twists, and specialized yoga positions.

A well-rounded core strength program stresses stability, flexibility, and endurance in addition to strength, creating a healthy and functioning core for everyday tasks and sports goals.

CHAPTER 1

Anatomy Of The Core

The core muscles serve as the body's powerhouse, contributing to stability, balance, and functional movement. Understanding these muscles' complexities is essential for good core strength training.

Understanding The Core Muscles And Their Functions

1. Rectus Abdominis: This muscle, sometimes known as the "six-pack," runs vertically across the front of the abdomen. Its major role is to bend the spine, which helps with exercises like crunches and sit-ups.

2. **Transverse Abdominis:** This muscle wraps around the sides and front of the abdomen like a corset. It stabilizes the spine and aids in core bracing, which is necessary for maintaining posture and supporting internal organs.

3. **Internal and external obliques:** These muscles on the sides of the abdomen allow for rotational and lateral flexion motions. They are also important in maintaining posture and stability.

4. **Erector Spinae:** A set of muscles that run down the spine, the erector spinae aids in spinal extension and upright posture.

5. **Multifidus:** These deep muscles provide stability and injury prevention by supporting the spine and assisting in rotating motions.

6. **Pelvic Floor Muscles:** These muscles at the base of the pelvis support the internal organs, help with posture, and are essential for urine and bowel control.

Exploring The Deep And Superficial Core Muscles

• **Deep Core Muscles:** These muscles, which include the transverse abdominis and multifidus, are located underneath the surface muscles and serve an important role in stabilization. They stabilize the spine and provide a firm foundation for movement when engaged during isometric activities.

• The rectus abdominis, external obliques, and erector spinae are more apparent and contribute to dynamic motions and torso flexion/extension.

Understanding how these muscles interact is critical in developing an effective core training regimen that activates and improves the whole core region.

CHAPTER 2

Benefits Of Core Strength Training

Improved Posture And Stability

The core muscles are essential for maintaining proper posture and stability. A strong core offers a firm foundation for the spine, assisting in optimal body support and alignment. Strengthening these muscles may help avoid slouching and lower back discomfort, enabling people to stand or sit more upright. Proper posture not only improves physical appearance but also decreases strain on muscles, joints, and ligaments, resulting in greater overall comfort.

Injury Prevention And Rehabilitation

A strong core reduces the likelihood of injury by providing stability and support to the whole body. When the core muscles are strong, the tension of ordinary motions is properly distributed, lessening the load on other muscle groups. Individuals with strong core muscles are also less likely to sustain injuries during physical activities or sports because they can better regulate their motions and maintain balance.

Furthermore, core strength training is often included in rehabilitation regimens for a variety of ailments. Core strength may help in recovery from back injuries, muscular strains, and other orthopedic issues. It aids in the rehabilitation of persons by restoring strength and stability.

Enhancing Athletic Performance

Core strength training is very beneficial to athletes in all sports. A strong core enhances agility, balance, and coordination, all of which are necessary for athletic success. It serves as a stable basis for producing power and moving energy between the upper and lower bodies, resulting in improved athletic ability.

A solid core, for example, provides for more efficient movement and helps athletes maintain good form when running, cycling, or swimming, minimizing fatigue and enhancing endurance. A strong core allows for faster and more controlled motions in sports that require rapid changes in direction or explosive movements.

In conclusion, the advantages of core strength training go well beyond merely getting a toned stomach. It's an important part of general fitness, as it helps with posture, injury prevention, and performance in a variety of physical activities.

CHAPTER 3
Core Strength Assessment

Before beginning a workout routine, it is critical to assess core strength. Understanding your starting point enables you to create individualized programs while also ensuring the safety and efficacy of your activities.

Self-Assessment Techniques

1. Core endurance may be determined by timing how long you can hold a plank. Maintain appropriate form while in the posture.

2. Core stability and control may be shown by balancing on one leg or utilizing balance boards.

3. Range of Motion Evaluation: Assessing the flexibility of the core muscles provides information about their condition.

4. Core Muscle Activation: Detecting muscle activation during certain actions or workouts aids in determining muscular strength.

Understanding Weaknesses And Imbalances

Identifying flaws or imbalances is critical. It might be obvious in a variety of ways:

• **Poor Posture:** Slouching or discomfort when sitting or standing may suggest a weakening in the core.

• **Lower Back Pain:** Consistent lower back pain may indicate a lack of core support.

• **Inefficient Movement Patterns:** Difficulties with particular motions or pain during workouts may indicate core weaknesses.

• **Asymmetry:** Distinctions in strength or flexibility between the left and right sides of the body may indicate an imbalance.

Understanding these factors allows you to adapt exercises, concentrating on particular regions that require growth while avoiding injuries.

Establishing a baseline via evaluation enables for customized training, gradually advancing toward efficiently and safely strengthening the core.

CHAPTER 4

Fundamental Core Exercises

The core encompasses the pelvic floor, obliques, lower back, and deep stabilizing muscles in addition to the abdominal muscles. Core strength isn't only about having nice abs; it's also about having functional strength and stability for everyday motions.

Exploring Isometric Exercises For Core Activation

Isometric workouts consist of contracting muscles without moving the joints. Planks are a great example since they engage the core without requiring too much movement. They aid in the development of endurance and steadiness, both of which are required for daily duties.

• **Plank Variations:** Side planks, forearm planks, and high planks all stimulate distinct core muscles and provide varied exercise.

Incorporating Planks And Variations

• **Side planks:** These work the obliques and increase lateral stability. Beginners might begin with a reduced side plank and work their way up.

• **Forearm Planks:** These exercises work the whole core, particularly the rectus abdominis and transverse abdominis.

It is critical for their efficiency that they maintain appropriate shape.

• **High planks:** These work the whole body, focusing on shoulder and arm strength as well as core stability.

Understanding The Role Of Breathing In Core Workouts

During core workouts, proper breathing patterns are critical. By stimulating the deep abdominal muscles and sustaining intra-abdominal pressure, diaphragmatic breathing helps to stabilize the core.

Effectiveness Hints

1. **Form vs. Duration:** Prioritize the form above duration. A well-executed 30-second plank outperforms a wobbly two-minute hold.

2. **Progression:** Gradually raise the difficulty to keep your core challenged. This may be accomplished by using longer holds, adding movement, or attempting advanced variants.

3. Consistency is essential. To observe increases in strength and stability, aim for a couple of core exercises each week.

4. **Rest and recovery:** Give your muscles time to recuperate.

Overworking the core without enough rest may result in injury or a plateau in development.

Individuals may develop a firm foundation for growing core strength, stability, and endurance, improving overall fitness, and lowering the risk of injury in everyday activities by learning basic core exercises such as planks and isometric holds.

CHAPTER 5

Dynamic Core Exercises

Incorporating Dynamic Movements For Core Strength

Core strength is more than simply holding static positions; it also entails mobility and stability during dynamic activities. Dynamic core workouts stimulate many muscles at the same time and often imitate real-life actions.

Discussing Russian Twists, Leg Raises, And Bicycle Crunches

1. Twists in Russia
Sit on the floor with your knees bent and your heels on the ground.

Lean gently back, maintaining your back straight. Hold a weight or a medicine ball in both hands. Tap the weight on the ground beside you as you rotate your body from side to side.

Russian twists improve rotational stability and strength while targeting the obliques, rectus abdominis, and transverse abdominis.

2. Leg Lifts

Lie down on your back, legs straight. Slowly raise your legs off the ground until they make a 90-degree angle, or as high as you can without arching your lower back. Lower them back down without letting them hit the floor.

Leg lifts develop the lower back muscles and stimulate the lower abdominals and hip flexors.

3. Crunches on a Bicycle

Lie on your back with your legs bent and your hands behind your head. Alternate between raising your left elbow to your right knee and stretching your left leg out. In a bicycling action, switch sides.

Bicycle crunches target the obliques and rectus abdominis, enhancing core stability and flexibility.

4. Variations on a Plank
Planks are essential for execution. Try side planks, plank jacks (jumping jack action

while holding a plank), or plank with shoulder taps to add dynamic components.

Plank variants not only exercise the whole core but also enhance endurance and stability in the muscles around the spine.

5. Climbers on Mount Everest

Start in a plank posture and work your way up. Bring one knee to your chest, then swiftly swap legs in a sprinting motion while maintaining your core engaged.

Mountain climbers train the whole core while also raising the heart rate, which has additional cardiovascular advantages.

6. Woodchoppers

Hold a weight or a medicine ball in both hands. Begin with the weight over one shoulder and work your way across your body and down to the opposing hip, engaging your core and twisting your torso.

The obliques, rectus abdominis, and shoulder muscles are targeted with woodchoppers, which simulate rotating motions utilized in everyday activity.

Dynamic core workouts aid in the development of functional strength, stability, and coordination. To avoid injuries and maximize the benefits of these workouts, always maintain perfect form and gradually increase intensity.

CHAPTER 6

Equipment-Based Core Workouts

A variety of equipment may greatly help core training, increasing both efficacy and variety in exercises. Here's how to use stability balls, resistance bands, and medicine balls to improve core strength and stability.

Using Stability Balls, Resistance Bands, And Medicine Balls

Balls of Stability

Stability balls, commonly referred to as Swiss balls or workout balls, provide a dynamic foundation for core training.

Their instability causes the core muscles to work harder.

Exercises:

• Ball Crunches: Do classic crunches on a ball, which increases engagement owing to the unstable surface.

• Plank on Ball: Raise your plank posture by resting your forearms on the ball, putting your core stability to the test.

• Bridge with Ball: While in a bridge posture, place your feet on the ball, activating the hamstrings and core at the same time.

Bands of Resistance

These elastic bands provide resistance to motions while also exercising core muscles throughout different activities.

Exercises:

• Pallof push: Holding the resistance band, standing sideways to a fixed point, and pushing away from the anchor, working core muscles against resistance.

• Standing Twist: Using both hands, twist your body from side to side, activating your obliques.

• Kneeling Woodchopper: Attach the band to a strong anchor and pull diagonally downwards to simulate a woodchopping action.

Medical Balls

Medicine balls give resistance and weight to workouts, boosting core stability and power.

Exercises:

• Russian Twists: Rotate your torso from side to side while holding the medicine ball, engaging your obliques.

• Medicine Ball V-Up: Perform a V-up movement while holding the ball between your feet, engaging both your upper and lower abdominals.

• Medicine Ball Slams: Raise the ball above and smash it down, activating the whole core and shoulders.

Exploring Advanced Core Training With Equipment

Combining equipment or incorporating unstable surfaces such as BOSU balls into advanced training can increase the complexity and intensity of exercises.

Exercises:

• BOSU Ball Plank: To engage stabilizing muscles, perform a plank on the unstable surface of a BOSU ball.

• Stability Ball Rollouts: Kneel with your hands on a stability ball and roll the ball forward while keeping your torso stable.

• Medicine Ball Push-Ups: Perform push-ups while holding a medicine ball, testing your balance and stability.

Understanding how to use equipment effectively in core workouts can significantly improve core strength, stability, and overall athletic performance by providing a variety of options for challenging and developing core muscles.

CHAPTER 7

Functional Core Training

Applying Core Strength To Daily Activities

The focus of functional core training is on how well your core muscles support daily movements. It consists of exercises that mimic real-life motions, improving your ability to perform daily tasks efficiently and safely.

1.   Core Stabilization Techniques: Techniques that focus on keeping the core stable during activities such as lifting groceries, carrying a child, or bending to tie shoelaces. Planks, bird dogs, and standing

core stabilization routines are examples of exercises.

2.   Core strength is important for maintaining proper posture while sitting or standing, which reduces strain on the spine and the risk of lower back pain.

3.   Balance and Coordination: Engaging core muscles improves balance and stability during activities requiring coordination, such as reaching for objects on high shelves or navigating uneven terrain.

Emphasizing Core Stability In Sports And Functional Movements

Functional core exercises have a significant impact on athletic performance. A strong core increases stability and power, which benefits a variety of activities:

1. **Running and jogging:** Core strength improves posture while running, reduces joint impact, and increases endurance.

2. **Weightlifting:** Maintaining form and stability during weightlifting exercises is critical for avoiding injuries and allowing for more controlled movements.

3.   Yoga and Pilates: Core stability is essential in these practices, allowing for better pose and movement execution.

Individuals can apply their strength to real-life situations by emphasizing functional core training, ensuring better performance, and lowering the risk of injury in a variety of activities.

CHAPTER 8

Core Training For Specific Goals

When it comes to core training, tailoring your exercises to specific goals can help you get the most out of them. Here are some examples of how core exercises can be used to achieve various goals:

Core Exercises For Weight Loss

Engaging the core is critical in weight loss efforts. It is critical to understand, however, that spot reduction is not a viable strategy for losing belly fat. Instead, core workouts increase overall calorie expenditure, promoting overall weight loss.

High-intensity interval training (HIIT) that incorporates core-centric exercises such as mountain climbers, planks, and burpees can help burn calories and increase metabolic rate. Compound movements that require core stabilization, such as squats, lunges, and deadlifts, also help to tone and slim the midsection.

Strengthening The Core For Back Pain Relief

Many cases of chronic back pain are the result of weak core muscles. By improving posture, and spinal stability, and reducing strain on the lower back, core strengthening can provide significant relief. Exercises that target the transverse abdominis, multifidus, and pelvic floor muscles are advantageous.

Bird dogs, bridges, and pelvic tilts, for example, help to stabilize the lumbar region. Yoga or Pilates, which focus on core engagement and flexibility, can also help relieve back pain.

Core Postnatal Rehabilitation

Women frequently experience weakened abdominal muscles after pregnancy as a result of the abdominal wall stretching during pregnancy. Postpartum core rehabilitation is critical for regaining strength and function. Gentle exercises like pelvic tilts, diaphragmatic breathing, and transverse abdominal activations are good starting points for regaining core stability. Gradually progressing to exercises such as modified planks and pelvic floor exercises aids in the restoration of core strength without putting the recovering body under strain.

Improving Sports Performance

Core strength is essential for athletic performance in a variety of sports. Swimmers, for example, require strong core muscles for stability and efficient stroke movements. Golfers rely on core stability in their swings for power and precision. Core workouts that are tailored to mimic sports-specific movements can improve performance. Rotational movements, anti-rotation exercises such as Pallof presses, and medicine ball throws can be used to simulate the demands of certain sports while strengthening the core.

Functional Fitness As A Whole

A strong core is essential for daily movements and activities. Functional core exercises are designed to mimic daily tasks, improving stability, balance, and overall functional fitness. Incorporating exercises such as farmer's walks, planks with limb motions, and stability ball exercises helps improve core strength for daily activities, lowering the risk of injury while doing actions such as lifting, bending, or reaching.

Understanding and tailoring core workouts to particular objectives ensures that exercises are useful and successful, resulting in targeted results as well as increased general fitness and health.

CHAPTER 9

Core Training Progressions

Gradual Advancement In Core Workouts

1.   Increasing Intensity Gradually: Gradually increasing the intensity and complexity of exercises is essential for continuous progress. Start with simple movements, then add resistance or leverage to enhance the workout.

2.   Adding Resistance: Incorporate resistance bands, weights, or other equipment into current routines, such as planks or Russian twists, to test the core muscles more.

3. Progressive Overload: As with any strength exercise, implementing the idea of progressive overload is crucial. It includes progressively increasing the tension put on the muscles to induce development and adaptability.

4. Increased repetitions or Sets: Incrementally increase the number of repetitions or sets completed for each exercise over time. This strategy aids in improving endurance and muscle strength.

5. Complex versions: Once skilled with fundamental maneuvers, go to more complex versions. For instance, go from basic planks to side planks or integrate motions like hanging leg lifts instead of ordinary leg raises.

Avoiding Plateaus And Maintaining Progress

1. Periodization: Implement a periodization strategy, which entails arranging exercises into periods. This strategy helps avoid plateaus by adjusting training factors like intensity, volume, or exercises.

2. Rest and healing: Adequate rest between workouts is vital for muscular healing and development. Alternate high-intensity core days with gentler, recovery-focused workouts to minimize burnout.

3. Constant Evaluation: Regularly review your progress, altering training programs appropriately.

Modify exercises, increase resistance, or modify workout formats if development stagnates.

4. Mixing Techniques: Incorporate a variety of isometric, dynamic, and equipment-based exercises to target diverse core muscles and prevent the body from adjusting to a certain regimen.

5. Cross-Training: Engage in activities beyond core-focused routines, such as swimming, cycling, or Pilates. These activities may complement core training and reduce boredom.

6. Core Strengthening Challenges: Challenge yourself frequently with focused core challenges, including maintaining a plank for an extended length or doing a

specified number of repetitions of hardcore exercises within a time constraint.

The Long-Term Approach

Sustainable improvement in core strength demands consistency, patience, and adaptability. Embrace the trip, modify as required, and celebrate milestones along the way. Remember, the aim is not only attaining a strong core but sustaining it over time for overall fitness and health.

CHAPTER 10

Integrating Core Training Into Your Routine

Designing A Comprehensive Core Workout Plan

Developing an effective core training routine requires numerous considerations:

1. Exercise Selection: Choose a range of exercises targeting various core muscles. Incorporate isometric, dynamic, and equipment-based workouts for a well-rounded regimen.

2. Progression: Start with fundamental exercises and progressively increase intensity to test your core.

Progression avoids plateaus and supports continued growth.

3. **Frequency:** Aim for regularity in training—2 to 3 times a week, allowing for proper recovery between sessions.

4. **Duration and Intensity:** Vary the duration and intensity of exercises to guarantee both endurance and strength development.

5. **Warm-up and cool-down:** To prepare the muscles, prioritize warming up with mild aerobic or dynamic stretches. Stretching after an exercise might help with healing.

6. Consistency is essential for long-term success. Better benefits come from sticking to your regimen.

Creating A Balanced Fitness Regimen Incorporating Core Strength

1. Cardiovascular Exercise: Combine core training with cardio exercises such as jogging, cycling, or swimming. This helps burn calories, improves general fitness, and strengthens the core.

2. Resistance Training: Include resistance workouts that target different muscle areas. Core strength and stability are supported by a strong overall body.

3. Stretching or yoga practices should be included to preserve flexibility. Muscle flexibility helps with core performance.

4. **Rest and recovery:** Allow enough time between exercises for muscles to heal and repair. Overtraining may stymie growth and raise the risk of injury.

5. **Nutrition:** A well-balanced diet promotes muscular development and recuperation. Adequate hydration and nutrient-dense meals contribute to overall fitness.

6. Prioritize mental health with activities such as meditation or mindfulness. Stress reduction has a good influence on physical performance.

By including core training in a comprehensive fitness plan, you lay a solid foundation for general health and performance.

Remember that perseverance and steady growth are essential for reaching your fitness objectives.

Conclusion

Accepting Core Strength Training For Long-Term Health

The basis of general fitness and wellness is core strength. We've recognized the importance of core muscles in maintaining our bodies and increasing functional motions as we've learned about them and trained them.

Considering The Importance Of Core Strength

We started our investigation by recognizing the importance of core strength beyond merely visual attractiveness. The core muscles, which include deep stabilizing muscles as well as superficial movers, serve as the body's center powerhouse, impacting almost every movement we make. Strengthening this region improves posture, balance, stability, and athletic performance while decreasing injury risk.

Promoting A Long-Term Commitment To Core Training

Building a strong core is a lifetime endeavor, not a one-time effort. We've learned the value of progression and variety in sustaining growth and minimizing plateaus as we've studied various exercises, dynamic movements, equipment-based routines, and functional training.

THE END